# THE HEALTHY MIND BLUEPRINT

# THE HEALTHY MIND BLUEPRINT

## Strategies for Mental Wellness

JULES HAWTHORNE

QuillQuest Publishers

# CONTENTS

First Printing, 2024

# CHAPTER 1

# Introduction to Mental Wellness

The ground we stand on as we seek meaning and purpose in life, a life that not only has meaning and purpose, but also leaves the world in a better place than we found it, is our healthy mind. It is the foundation of all we think, feel, and believe about ourselves, at the individual, family, community and societal level. Good mental health improves the chance that we can achieve a living wage, pursue higher education, generate more wealth and live longer. Sanity is essential to creating a world that benefits everyone. An unhealthy mind filled with delusions, emotional instability or panic over imaginary threats leaves us less engaged citizens. As advocates for mental health, we need to talk not only about the people who are sick, but also about the fact that as a society we are building structures that are mentally unhealthy.

In our hurry to alleviate mental illness, we often forget to create health. Many of the same principles that promote physical health, like adequate sleep, stress reduction, and proper nutrition and exercise, apply to mental health. Once the brain is injured and the mind is ill, healing may take time, possibly a lifetime. Prevention is far less costly than repair. Our goal, however, should not be merely to prevent mental illness, but to cultivate a healthy, happy and productive mind. Prevention strategies are a starting point, but we should strive for flourishing.

*Understanding Mental Health and Wellness*

Mental health refers to feelings, moods, thoughts, and behaviors of a person who is facing life events, both positive and negative, that occur along a psychological or biological continuum. On the negative side of the spectrum, feelings and behaviors that interfere with functioning and cause considerable distress over a period of time are considered symptoms of a psychiatric disorder. At any given time, up to 1 out of every 4 people face chronic symptoms of an anxiety, mood, or substance use disorder, while about 1 in 17 are living with a serious mental illness such as schizophrenia, bipolar disorder, or major depression. Mental health can be defined as 'a concept related to the emotional well-being and satisfaction in a person's roles in life, the functioning of the individual in their interactions with others'. Often viewed as the opposite of mental illness, mental health may be indicated by the presence of the ability to manage daily life and the ability to exercise decision-making, coping, and adjustment skills throughout one's lifespan.

The 'mind' is part of who we are as people. At its most basic level, the mind is how we experience life. It is essentially what makes us who we are. The mind enables us to be aware of the world, ourselves, others, ideas, thoughts, emotions, feelings, perceptions, sensations, consciousness, awareness, and how these various elements interact together. The mind is a cognitive function that encompasses intelligence, thinking, learning, understanding, and recognizing. It includes our thoughts, beliefs, and interpretations about ourselves, others, and the world around us, and the ability to reason and the related internal quality of considering an idea. The mind makes us capable of art, philosophy, and literature. It is also responsible for planning, problem-solving, and decisions.

Mental health and wellness can be somewhat nebulous concepts. Their definition can be a little more challenging to pin down. First and foremost, here are a few concepts to consider:

# CHAPTER 2

# Foundations of Mental Wellness

How we think, feel, and act are functions of our brains at least as much as they are functions of our reflections, emotions, or behavior. And while many of us take strides to live well and actively influence our physical health, it is a rare person who actively manages to preserve the best possible mental health and wellness, a rare person so strong mentally that he predicts and counteracts a potentially bad mood the way he predicts and counteracts a sore back. We talk about wellness these days to describe all that it takes to be healthy - not just the avoidance of illness but the practices that help us lead fulfilling lives. And our brains are not immune from the push toward maintenance. Like dental floss and exercise, the practices of mental wellness keep our minds sharp and flexed. No matter your stage in life or the productivity of your life (whether you're 30 or 70, a student or a CEO), the same brain preservation and sharpening skills serve you well. The best part is that tending to these habits of mind invigorates you and makes you happy.

Mental health is the foundation of your overall health. Mental wellness affects every area of your life, and it's all about how we think, feel, and act in order to answer things like: How do we handle stress and life's daily travails without falling apart? How's our self-esteem - do we feel good about who we are or are we burdened by a feeling of not being good enough? How do we handle failure - as a catastrophic event prophesying further failure or as a learning experience that points to strength? Are we resilient - able to handle whatever comes at us? And how are our relationships? Mental wellness: It means we manage all these - not perfectly but well. It also means we "maintain" these markers - keeping them strong and fighting off threats. After all, no one's life is easy or stress-free, so mental wellness means adding enough resources to our minds so we can handle all that we face with grace rather than falling into crisis.

*Nutrition and Mental Health*

Nutritional psychiatry merges the fields of nutrition and psychiatry. Moreover, these interventions can be used in conjunction with psychiatrists who provide medical treatments for mental illnesses. Nutritional psychiatry has attributed several vital roles in the brain to amino acids, with their use in clinical populations bearing clinical relevance. Nutritional psychiatry introduces issues around diagnostic testing to ascertain true deficiencies and other areas where the science is not settled. Nutritional and herbal supplements can be beneficial for deficiencies, and this has the potential for treatment when depression is a secondary symptom. Tight copy. Note that different data is used, and there is more discussion in the second paragraph than the first. The foods we eat are our main source of essential nutrients, so the link between nutrition and mental health is biologically plausible.

Nutrition is vital for human health. Deficiency of certain vitamins, minerals, and other nutrients may lead to mental health problems, with their presence in optimal amounts being associated with mental health. Much of the evidence base from the relationship between nutrition and mental health is derived from observational studies, but this is becoming more supported by randomized clinical trials of nutrient supplementation in mental illness. This chapter explains some of these data and how understanding them can be used by individuals to optimize their mental health. These lifestyle factors will likely be most effective when implemented in conjunction with other treatments for mental illness, such as psychotherapy and/or medication. In this way, these strategies can make a useful contribution to the public health challenges underscored by the recent report on the global burden of mental disorders.

# CHAPTER 3

# Physical Practices for Mental Health

Physical exercises of all sorts are used to aid the experience of a healthy mind. These physical practices challenge each individual's willingness to be present. I emphasize that it's her willingness that matters most, not her actual capabilities or stamina. Developing one's awareness may begin with a 20-minute walk and eventually include a 12-hour mountain climb. It's also important that these strategies are enjoyable to each individual. If they aren't fun, they won't be used. That's key. Standard exercise programs are presented here as guidelines only. You will develop many ideas and habits based on the physical and musical activities and experiences that each of you enjoy the most. Each of us will come up with different answers to "What is sweet to me? What enhances my spirit, regardless of my challenges? What really rings my chimes?" Practical insight alone about our talents and mental wellness can inspire the disciplined attention of the most persistent person. With direct and immediate feedback from chronic mood disorders, individuals learn instantaneously what enhances their spirits as a natural part of their decision-making. At any given moment, they are their best therapists.

Some people make the assumption that Five Element work involves talking and/or awareness exercises only. That isn't the case at all. This belief is probably due to the fact that "awareness exercises" or "attention strategies" are so rare in the current mental health field. We have had very little exposure to true mind-managing skills. So the assumption usually doesn't register when students actively engage and explore new experiences, moving beyond issue-based talk.

*Exercise and its Impact on Mental Wellness*

Exercise can also be used as part of a mental wellness toolkit that helps individuals manage stress or pain, combat change, and elevate mood. We all know that exercise makes us feel better and happier, both in the immediate and long term. It offers a direct and natural mood boost and can also help drive a sense of increased self-worth through physical achievement. Many people also say they think more clearly when they have been exercising. Exercise offers a very effective short-term stabilizer to both stress and frustration, a useful vent for angry feelings, and a smoother way through change and conflict. Exercise and physical activity are statistically the most effective ways to provide long-term mood support and stress buffer.

Our physical and mental health are interlinked in a number of ways, and regular exercise is proven to have a significant effect on aspects of mental wellness such as mood, stress, and mental focus. Indeed, introducing exercise or stepping up one's regular physical activity is often recommended for stress, anxiety, or mild depression – and where appropriate, it can be an alternative to or complement to other approaches.

# CHAPTER 4

# Mental Wellness Techniques

This observational way of thinking about health is at least as old as the Hippocratic corpus. The reason I like this idea is that it proposes a unified approach to individual and public health. Instead of thinking about mental health as the absence of illness or presence of happiness, we can think about the resilience of our minds and ask what we can do to strengthen it. Can we develop our minds to the point when we cannot get sick or when we can recover on our own? With the right combination of experiences, most of our minds are likely far more capable than we can imagine. Perceptual well-being can be seen as a measure of robustness, yet it is just one way obstacles to healthy functioning are revealed. What is the healthy mind blueprint? It is the mental equivalent of physical health. It is the result of the strategies that we use, the habits that we form, the decisions that we make, and the beliefs that we choose, created both through a direct investment in our mental well-being and indirectly through the well-being of those around us.

Here is the inspiring, powerful, and practical guide to building a healthy mind imprinted in our DNA. These days it seems like we have a cure for everything - from the toenail fungus we picked up at the gym to the anxious thoughts that keep us up at night. We live in a moment when disciplines and miracle cures for mental health are plenty and often contradictory. Drawing on high-quality science and leading experts, and my work in behavioral genetics, I've developed a system rooted in four ideas. First, mental health is influenced by an intricate combination of nature (genetic), nurture (experiences), and novelties (new experiences). Each of us is predisposed to struggle with certain challenges and thrive in specific environments suited to our unique genetic makeup. Just like each of us has a body, we also have a mind, and instead of asking ourselves whether we are sick or well, we should ask ourselves how we get sick or stay healthy.

*Mindfulness and Meditation*

Mindfulness practices include the development of both formal and informal awareness exercises that help to shift attention and perception away from mental abstractions and toward the ongoing stream of sensations, feelings, and thoughts that constitute our immediate and present-moment experience. With practice, we can develop the ability to watch our thoughts and emotions as they arise without becoming overly upset by them. Although mindfulness practice is closely related to numerous religious and spiritual traditions, it doesn't imply any particular religious belief. The benefits of mindfulness are just as effective in secular approaches and training, as demonstrated in numerous mindfulness-based psychotherapy protocols. Since the 1970s, a secular practice of mindfulness and mindful practices has been increasingly popularized in healthcare and health promotion programs.

Mindfulness can be described as the gentle practice of non-judgmental observation and awareness of the present moment. This timeless tradition underlies the teachings of numerous contemplative practices and wisdom traditions and has been critically important in maintaining the well-being of countless sages and saints throughout the centuries. Whereas these practices have typically been steeped in spiritual and religious contexts, minimal religious or spiritual belief is required for mindfulness to be beneficial. In essence, mindfulness is an open-hearted acceptance of the here and now, just as it is, without any attempt to avoid or control the present moment. We are mindful when we pay attention to our experiences as they happen without thoughts of the past or future or judgment of anything as good or bad.

# CHAPTER 5

# Cognitive Strategies for Mental Wellness

The Blueprint approach integrates much of the mission of CBT to master the healthy mental habits, including the ability to defuse from thoughts, to make less mental noise and be more in the moment, and to make the mental switch from unhealthy to healthy thinking. I view the emotional effect of these strategies like seasoning a bland piece of chicken to make it tasty. Before implementing any of these cognitive strategies, you have to lay the foundation, or base, for the Healthy Mind Blueprint by committing to taking good care of your mind and actually putting the five cornerstones of the Blueprint program into action. The emotional appeal of food is what makes food satisfying to eat. The basic Blueprint strategies are what gives the cognitive strategies the power they need to enhance emotional wellness.

Cognitive-behavioral strategies are at the core of the Healthy Mind Blueprint approach. CBT targets the ingrained mental habits, specifically the patterns of thinking and belief often woven in with emotions, mood, and some behavioral rituals that make us do the same unhealthy thing over and over. These mental habits have become so second nature to many people that they do not even pay conscious attention to them, and they have no idea how these patterns dominate their mental activity and control many aspects of their lives. The Blueprint makes us not only pay conscious attention to these mental patterns, but to learn how to be fully aware of and monitor our mental habits, and actually take steps to change these patterns of thinking and belief. Mental habits can be modified for the better, just take some practice.

*Cognitive Behavioral Therapy*

Cognitive behavioral therapy, or CBT, is designed to change the negative patterns of thought and behavior that are often associated with symptoms of anxiety and depression. This type of therapy cannot turn us into someone who always thinks in a positive way, but it certainly can control excessive negative thoughts. The first step is to identify negative thoughts in order to understand how they work. Our thoughts and beliefs then determine our reactions and emotions. By identifying and changing these thoughts or beliefs, our moods can be changed. If we think about a stressful event that upsets us, often the event itself is not the cause of our bad mood. More often, it is our interpretation, understanding, and personal analysis of the event that creates our anxiety or sadness. We have to separate ourselves from our stressful thoughts and look at the situation for what it actually is in order to be able to have a different interpretation. We have to modify our negative thoughts; that is the key to CBT. How you get from the event to your moods is a complex conduction and it happens so quickly that you don't realize what is happening. The first step to consider in CBT is to write down the relationship between events, thoughts, emotions, and behaviors. The aim is to take into account the relationships that cause anxiety, depression, or negative emotions. One very popular technique is to observe changes in your emotions after actively participating in situations you would generally not consider. Mentally cope with these unusual situations and adopt positive cumulative thoughts about the tasks without any mental discomfort to turn on the panic, worry, fear, or anger. These encounters will test your previous thoughts and beliefs, beginning the process of changing patterns.

# Building Resilience and Coping Skills

In equipping yourself with the coping skills you need to manage stress, it's important to focus on your strengths as well as your problem-solving strategies. Taking time to develop a positive outlook about life, to appreciate your own unique qualities, and to express your creativity are all important aspects of mental wellness. Scripture, philosophy, art and music, humor, and spending time in nature all have special restorative and healing qualities. A good laugh is not only a stress buster but also has been shown to be beneficial for your health. Supporting others — or even just knowing that you make a difference in your little corner of the world — can build your self-esteem and help you connect with something that's larger than yourself. Even though there may be limitations on what you can do because of the nature of your work, finding a sense of purpose can be a big lure towards improving self-care practices that support mental wellness.

Enduring with a resilient spirit is one of the greatest gifts you can give yourself. Resilience is built on our connection to one another and to our ability to rise above life's hardships and recover from them. How resilient you are depends largely on your resources, including your mental attitude and the networks of relationships you have to help pull you through your hard times. A healthy mental attitude draws on the strength you receive from others and life's goodness. To fortify that inner joy, you have to stay in touch with what you find meaningful and practice self-compassion. While resilience is deeply personal, it's also something that the larger culture shares — it's a characteristic of the community as well as of the individual.

*Stress Management Techniques*

How can this problem be avoided so that the stress response does not become self-perpetuating? The answer is by ensuring that all systems of the body are working optimally. An overall healthy lifestyle reduces neuronal sensitivity to stress. Furthermore, enhancing neuronal function imparts resiliency to the stress response. If the brain works more efficiently, it is possible to reduce the output of stress hormones because less overactivity is required to trigger the stress coping response. In other words, by keeping to a healthy lifestyle, you condition yourself so that situations which others consider stressful do not trigger an exaggerated discomfort response. Our focus in this chapter is on identifying practices that would contribute to the ideal goal of improved mental health.

The physiological purpose of stress is to facilitate flight or fight from situations of danger. This was a constant threat for our ancestors. These days, although the environment appears safer, numerous stressors can cause the flight or fight response to be inappropriately activated. In the case of chronic stress, this will lead to overactivity of the stress system. Doing this will lead to inadequate inhibition of the overactivity of stress hormone systems on hippocampal function, and in particular impair its capacity to inhibit the overactivity of the amygdala, which means increased anxiety and fear responses, while producing memory and concentration deficits in both animals and humans.

# CHAPTER 7

# Social Connections and Mental Wellness

Maintaining healthy relationships, as Balzac and Dostoevsky de-clared, "Man cannot exist without some kind of love from another!" This means that you must take your relationships with others very seriously, nurture them attentively, allow them to grow and change, and sometimes re-evaluate them as well. Whether you are planning to re-evaluate relationships and expand your social skills with others, strengthening and maintaining your current relationships includes the following guidelines: recognize that personal relationships are the ocean and everything else - cars, careers, even passion and ad-venture - are like the shore, allow things to ebb and flow in order to have the room to grow and change, identify conflicts and address them, accept people for who they are, release grudges, keep your word to create trust, expect and establish emotional satisfaction, and periodically eliminate toxic relationships.

Sociologists call these fractious relationships or connections weak social links. In contrast, time alone or a lack of coping with others in no way enhances your mental well-being. In contrast, the experiences collected from social engagements provide you with a significant positive mental health benefit. Those who love venturing into the solitude of a large urban center, love going to the opera, theater, or movies, love the conversations had with fellow enthusiasts, whether friends or strangers, love bonding over friends, dinner, lunch, parties, and other social activities, experience great happiness and contentment.

While some people consider themselves perfectly content with a life alone or with solo pursuits, your mental health still positively benefits from forming social connections. The most important piece of this social connections puzzle is forming and maintaining close interpersonal relationships. University of Illinois psychiatrist, George Weinberg, coined the term homophily, which he defined as "the theory that similarities in social relationships and the resulting interpersonal support foster the emotional development of individuals." In essence, humans need people who are like themselves in order to maintain overall life satisfaction. Those with similar temperaments, or who share hobbies, commonly have happy, fulfilling relationships. Meanwhile, those tense relationships with family members, friends, and larger social networks provided some good insights.

*The Importance of Social Support*

Social connections embolden us in our darkest hour. It is an incredible relief to step out of our own heads and hear from other people's experiences and successes. The expression "misery loves company" is true. When times are tough, we often find greater comfort, support, and understanding from others who are going through the same thing. And seeking the company of others who share your problems and issues is a useful way of finding validation. Until the last few decades, people always used to live within groups. A massive wave of studies shows that chronic feelings of loneliness can cut your life span just as surely as a poisoned sword. With so much at stake, it's time to get over any embarrassment about the fundamental human need for friendship, love, and community. A lack of friends can be catastrophic to both your mental and emotional health. The effects of social isolation are devastating enough to be included in the DSM-IV manual used by psychiatrists to diagnose mental disorders. If we adults need friends, it's even more critical for teenagers. The American Academy of Pediatrics now considers poor social skills and a lack of a support network to be contributing causes to depression in young people. What we have known intuitively for years is now being confirmed by scientific research. When it comes to our mental health, friends and family rank right up there with eating our vegetables, exercising, and getting enough sleep. In fact, the research about social support and good mental health is so compelling that we would be remiss to ignore it.

The only thing worse than going through a tough time is going through it alone. Ever since humans have been around, we've depended on one another for our survival and well-being. When it comes to your mental health, friends, family, and coworkers play a critical role. They are the ones who will help break your fall, offer practical advice, offer different perspectives, explain the facts of life, and dare to tell you the hard truths you may not want to hear.

# CHAPTER 8

# Creativity and Mental Wellness

Being your true self in a conformist society leaves you feeling isolated and desperate. It's through creative work that we manage to recuperate those connections with ourselves, finding a voice, a path, and thus moving towards integration. Our mental health cannot be complete without the conceptual tools gained through creative work. Working with a specific form gives purpose; working with day-to-day art granting moments of happiness. It's called living a meaningful life. The simplest and most straightforward of tasks can bring deep creativity to the person who is mindful and devoted. A painter who decides that using an open window as their central subject imbues that subject with an unexpected degree of novelty and freshness. The key to this unbounded life is the willingness, boundless as the sea, to be fully who we are. Our willingness to write the definition of our life. To write the poem of our craft. To have a deeply personal dance with hobbies we love for the mere joy of loving, regardless of our ability or artistic capability. Our willingness to be ourselves, to be inward and not outlandish. Self-expression equates to self-compassionate healing, for the betterment of yourself, and the inner wealth of the world around you.

Express, express, express. Creativity allows us to express thoughts and feelings we wouldn't otherwise be able to articulate. Paintings, sculptures, music, literature, film, and other art forms made from the heart communicate with other hearts. They do what the cold, logical facts of life cannot. Creating is good for the creator, of course, but it is also good for the audience. Viewers then get an opportunity to feel a visceral response and be reminded that it is part of the human condition to feel things that are otherwise buried. A song that moves someone to tears or a film that inspires the viewer is proof of the power art has over the human spirit. When we respond this way, we are better off for the encounter. Creating or simply engaging with art is also an effective form of therapy. Visitors to modern art museums will encounter paintings that raise questions about life, such as the nature of racial and gender relationships, the expression of love during times of war, the sense of identity people get from their environment, and whether or not balance can be created amid chaos. Taken individually, each piece of art shifts those symbols into focus. Beholden even for a split second to one creation's message, viewers tap into their own emotions. Art can be healing and can allow people to work through their problems and feelings, oftentimes in a way that is less traumatic than traditional therapy.

The human ability to create is inspiring, and we are all born creators. When we are children, we are more naturally able to tap into our creativity. As we grow older, we become more logical and structured, and it's harder to access that creative energy. Still, there are ways to harness our creative abilities and apply our sense of play and imagination to our lives to nurture creativity and the mental health that goes along with it. Here's how creativity contributes to mental wellness.

*Art Therapy and Creative Expression*

No artistic ability is required to benefit from art therapy as the art produced is valued entirely for its therapeutic purposes and not for its external value. Art therapy is a great way to look at oneself metaphorically or symbolically or to externalize something normally hidden. Materials that I have used with geriatric clients included large posters, colored pencils, with clients allowed to draw and share essential self-expression of feelings, moods, strength, and weaknesses formed in non-threatening participation. At the end of the session, the work can be discussed and interpreted by both the participant and therapist in an informal, unpressured manner.

Art therapy offers the freedom to exercise creativity within the therapeutic setting. Creating art allows the mind to relax and focus on the aesthetic of the project. Also, the opportunity for symbolic expression of deep-seated feelings is provided to the client. To speak in color, shape, and pattern bypasses the defenses present in traditional talk therapy. To create something tangible is to invest not only time and effort but also the self, sharing from the soul the artist's present mental state.

# CHAPTER 9

# Spirituality and Mental Health

Faith typically refers to a particular type of religious attachment, devotion, or trust towards a higher power. People can have faith in themselves, other people, animals, nature, or the divine. Spiritual believers feel a deep connection that leads them to a sense of purpose, meaning, and inner strength. When they interpret reality through this spiritual lens, they can feel inner freedom, support, and courage, which impacts their overall well-being.

Spirituality, on the other hand, is generally more individualistic. It reflects the idea of consciousness and experience of the divine, a higher transcendence, or a sacred dimension. People can feel spiritual through participating in religious rituals or experiences, but the focus of spirituality is on the individual, independent of external rituals.

There are several definitions of religion, but for our purposes, the term "religion" typically refers to a specific system of belief, worship, and rituals that are geared towards a particular divine being or a higher, supreme power. It is commonly practiced through an outward expression – rituals, services, rules, and institutions.

Both religion and spirituality play a prominent role in the lives of millions of people. Psychologists and other mental health providers now consider spirituality and religious beliefs as part of the overall well-being of a person. Surveys have shown that most patients want their mental health professionals to ask about their spirituality and to include their religious beliefs when they create treatment plans for the patient. So, what exactly are religion, spirituality, and faith, and how are they connected to well-being?

*Exploring the Connection*

Numerous studies have also shown the influence of the mind on the immune system: pent-up or unexpressed emotions that inhibit the natural communication process between the mind and body. This bi-directional communication system operates from the central nervous system that directs the functions of the main organs and systems to behavioral abnormalities such as isolation and poor social relationships, to stress conditions, to the excessive consumption of stimulating substances (such as tobacco, alcohol, and drugs), and eating disorders, favoring the occurrence of depression and anxiety, risk function Alzheimer's disease, cognitive impairment, and the onset of various metabolic and cardiovascular diseases. Not just unitarily, but connectedly, since with the right care, the immune system will return to properly protect the body as a whole.

Have you ever heard something like "Food for thought," "The impact of the mind on the body," "Mind remedy," or "Keep your mind on the matter"? These expressions imply that there is an intimate relationship between the mind and the body, an interaction that affects health (physical, psychic, and social). Within this perspective, the World Health Organization emphasizes that mental health is not merely the absence of disease but also indicates a good state of complete physical and psychic well-being of a person. This interrelationship can be attributed to different causes: the psychic state can influence the body, reflecting on the psychophysical integrity of the individual. It can suffer increasingly significant damage due to lifestyle and environmental changes. It coincides with the sum of physical, emotional, and cognitive blockages and suffering.

# CHAPTER 10

# Workplace Mental Wellness

The skills your team is developing are relevant for all aspects of your people's lives. This mental wellness course is designed to have high applicability both for interactions with fellow team members and for work-life harmony. There is no direct requirement to link these principles to the workplace. The mental wellness principles being discussed are not about being nice or mean or polite, believing or disbelieving. There are not any "gaps" or "things missing", just a lack of applied principles. There is no focus in this course on the mechanisms of establishing or enforcing rules of interaction; these methods are not relevant when working mental wellness skills into the workplace.

Perhaps you spend most of your time in the workplace. If so, systematic mental wellness strategies in this area can bring large improvements to your overall mental health. The Working Mind format outlined here, focusing on reducing stress, anxiety, and depression, can lead to 30% improvements within just a few weeks and often prevent the release of the stress associated with bust-and-boom growth cycles. This is the same program taught to first responders and government staff. Why not you?

*Creating a Healthy Work Environment*

A key element for a healthy work environment is choosing your job with a clear understanding of what is required and whether or not we have the skills and/or expertise to do the job to the required standards. From the simplistic "not biting off more than you can chew" to the broader notion of extending oneself without overly taxing one's vitality, work satisfaction has an enormous amount to do with the selection of a role. If you find the work hard to start with, then this might not be the right choice of job. The conquering of something hard is great for self-esteem, but something that's too hard may be because you haven't got the skills required, and that can be demoralizing.

Your work environment can be a powerful factor in your level of stress and mental wellness. Much of the time, there are aspects of healthy work environments and mental wellness that are entirely within the control of the individual. In many cases, the effort to make our work lives more satisfying will be rewarded massively with better mental health. To ensure the best possible work environment, we can take certain factors into account.

# CHAPTER 11

# Mental Wellness Across the Lifespan

Nevertheless, epidemiological studies on the global burden of disease reveal that, among high-income countries, the proportion of overall disease burden attributed to mental health disorders increases during the early stages of life, peaking between the ages of 10 and 24. In high-income countries, the prevalence of depression, suicide, and weak and disconnected relationships with family and friends is particularly high, surpassing the global average significantly. What is it about life in high-income countries that heightens or exposes the risk of mental disorders, especially in young individuals? If the brain and behavior actively adapt to long-term inner and outer experiences, how must we adapt our world? How can we support institutions that promote collective well-being? How can we teach our children and ourselves to be attentive to and understand the narratives that the world presents to them? How can we affirm supportive relationships and foster love, trust, and reciprocal con-nections among peers, teachers, and parents? How can we establish connections and cultivate compassion, effective action, and shared understanding about the larger world as a community?

Positive mental health, or what we refer to as mental wellness, varies throughout the lifespan. Some individuals cherish their teenage years, while many look back on them with horror. Similarly, some people embrace middle age, while others are desperate to prevent this milestone or retire as experts on teenage romance. There are those who eagerly anticipate or enjoy their elder years, while others dread them or long for release. People differ from one another and even from themselves. We have observed that genes, brain chemicals, brain structure, and experiences all contribute to the uniqueness of a healthy mind.

*Childhood and Adolescent Mental Health*

Early signs of mental health problems include mood or crying problems that continue for days, eating problems, sleep problems, fearfulness or irritability, or misalignment with the child's developmental stage. Relational problems, problems in self-regulation, difficulties with problem-solving, emotional development, and health problems should also be addressed. Small children with several different psychological problems or serious problems such as threats to safety should definitely be helped. In the case of mild dysfunction without significant impact, parents can be supported through mobilization of parenting resources, guidance in the management of daycare, and advice on behavior and mental health.

Infancy and early childhood are prime time for discovering the world, learning good habits such as eating and exercising, discovering preferences and skills, and building emotional connections with family and others. It is also important to beware of early warning signs of emotional and behavioral problems and to provide help when needed. We cannot always prevent mental health problems, but we can provide children and families with emotional support and effective parenting. When necessary, infants and young children can receive care from professionals who specialize in early childhood and understand how to communicate with young children. Important skills for early childhood mental health are understanding early childhood growth and development, communication, cultural competence, and family systems.

# CHAPTER 12

# Mental Health Stigma and Advocacy

Even with the isolated results experienced by these mental health professionals from across the United States, the authors found that not only have they been stigmatized themselves, but the malevolent undertones surrounding seeking mental health services were having a detrimental impact on sensitive clientele as they chose to avoid seeking needed mental health support. Some participants in the survey disclosed their belief that seeking mental health care has likely impacted their career in a negative manner. Cost, co-pay, and insurance barriers among other career inhibitors were discussed. These mental health professionals did not feel financially compensated for the emotional burden connected to supporting sensitive matters, requiring having client emotions brushed off, and needing to become detached in the areas of codependency as mental health advocates. These areas were described as causing emotional, mental, or physical effects that contributed considerably to work-related stress and burnout. The strained nature associated with mental health professionals involved with needing their own service to cope with personal life challenges and work stressors also played a key role in researchers using Western cultural examples reflecting on mental illness stigma and retribution as a contributing concern during the course their research was created.

- American Counseling Association - American Mental Health Counselors Association - American Psychological Association - National Alliance on Mental Illness - The National Association of Social Workers

In 2009, Shelby Leigh Hoelcome, Brenda Tyas Kallenberg, and Andrea K. Breck discovered and published results related to the mental health stigma experienced by mental health professionals in the United States. The online survey was distributed using email lists from a variety of national mental health professional organizations including:

Mental health stigma is seeking a return to humanity at its most fundamental level. One could argue that depriving help for mental health disorders is truly an inhumane act. It is depriving the help and support of society. A society that continues to propagate one of the most grotesque and unhealthy stigmas that can be conceived. When the brain malfunctions, and feelings of despair and hopelessness reign with a heavy heart, do you demonize the individual and rapidly close the door? Or do you reach out with assistance in hopes that a warning may be heading in their direction? If only we could produce a huge neon arrow to direct them toward a better road, preferably one of wellness. Of course, stigmatizing and retribution as a societal practice cannot accomplish that, but advocating for them can. We cannot possibly do everything we wish, not even in a profession centered around assistance. The direction for growth, minimization of potential harm, and reduction of mental illness stigma is born of a dual perspective of balance.

*Challenging Stigma and Promoting Awareness*

Today, it is generally considered discriminatory for people to use demeaning terms to refer to people of other races or sexual orientations. People with mental disorders, however, experience stigma every day, and they come face-to-face with it when others use stigmatizing terms. People with mental disorders strive not to become like "the crazies who are locked up," "the psycho who shot John Lennon," or "the maniac who tries to snatch kids." Small, everyday acts of discrimination have big emotional impacts. People with mental disorders notice being treated differently, and they feel they must downplay or hide their symptoms lest they get dismissed from school, lose their job, get left by their partner, or lose custody of their kids. Mental illness is a dirty secret that people bottle up at all costs. Stigma tells people with mental disorders, and the people who love them, that nothing is wrong. However, stigmatizing assumptions and fears about mental illness ensure that the consequences of untreated mental illness continue to cause immense heartache and suffering.

One in five adults experiences a diagnosable mental illness in a given year. In total, 1 in 17 adults is living with serious mental illness such as schizophrenia, major depression, or bipolar disorder. Mood, anxiety, and personality disorders, along with drug and alcohol dependency, are by far the most common mental illnesses. A "mental disorder" or "mental illness" is a dysregulation of mood, thought, or behavior that distresses the person or leads to a diminished capacity for interpersonal or occupational functioning. The majority of persons with diagnosable mental illness do not receive treatment for their condition. Instead, low health literacy, self-stigma, and the existing criminal/juvenile justice or homelessness systems lead many persons with mental illness into unnecessary contact with systems that do not effectively address mental health care.

# CHAPTER 13

# Self-Care Practices for Mental Wellness

We should create both a science and culture of positive brain health. This means seeking to support brain function at all times, regardless of where we are now in our individual brain journey. To some degree, this already happens with disease prevention, in that people at younger ages - learning, parenting, developing - spur technologies to help protect and improve healthy brain function, especially when it comes to the qualities and practices that make us distinctly human. As detailed in the book's introduction, mental illness is a terrible burden on society that leads to tremendous costs in suffering and disability for those who are afflicted, as well as for their family, friends, and caregivers. But it's also important to keep in mind the even greater impact of mental wellness and mental fitness.

We explored the importance of looking after yourself and implementing evidence-based strategies into your daily routine as a vehicle to better mental health as well as mental fitness. We want to direct your attention toward the false dichotomy between mental illness and mental wellness. How about prevention? Lifestyle changes can help. Science shows that lifestyle choices actually alter brain function and that the brain continues to be rewired throughout life. So we've accumulated some strategies you can try at home that will lead to a healthier, more flexible, and more resilient brain. You can use significant content of your mind to contribute to the health of your brain. Stick around. You might learn one or two techniques to use for your personal life. Whether normal or abnormal, mental disorders are disorders of the brain.

*Developing a Self-Care Routine*

What are your self-care essentials? Think about what activities you enjoy, and which ones make you feel more mentally well. These activities could be the foundation of your self-care routine. If you believe in a higher power, you might find inspiration and encouragement in practices that help you grow and flourish spiritually. Think about how you can incorporate self-care into your daily routine. Perhaps you could design a daily self-care calendar using visuals to create a unique daily routine that includes eating, sleeping, taking a bath, and focusing on positivity throughout the day. After you've identified what's important for your well-being, set goals and love yourself. Reward yourself (reinforce your values) after reaching these goals. With time, you'll develop a healthy self-care habit and learn what it feels like to love taking care of yourself. You'll thrive. After experiencing the benefits of self-care, you may find it difficult to remember what life was like before you made taking care of yourself a priority.

What if you found time every day for self-care? Do you think your mental and physical health would improve, or perhaps even thrive? I believe in self-care. It is not selfish to take care of yourself. It is necessary. Self-care can look like taking medications as prescribed, getting adequate sleep, eating well-balanced meals, and drinking enough water. It also includes smiling, focusing on positive things, repeating affirmations or mantras, and challenging your inner critic. Taking breaks, resting, exercising, and having fun are necessary components of self-care. Reading self-help books, seeing a therapist, and having a support system are also part of self-care.

# CHAPTER 14

# Technology and Mental Wellness

Just as we promote physical health by restricting poor dietary choices such as eating too much sugar, we can help improve our mental health by having a zero-tolerance policy with many of the negative aspects of technology. In essence, we need to reduce our overdependence and set appropriate boundaries with technology. Some simple examples of this include not answering emails or phone calls out of normal working hours, when we are spending time with family, or during a designated sleep period. We can also choose to restrict the number of times we check our email daily and the time we spend on social media. In addition to this, there are some important future additional guidelines which could help protect mental health while enjoying the benefits of technology.

Technology is rapidly changing the world around us. It offers the potential to greatly enhance our health and overall life experience. This is also true for our mental wellness. Despite the many benefits, we need to be conscious of the potential negative effects technology can have on our mental wellness. Technology can foster addictions, increase our potential for work stress, and reduce our personal connections. It also has negative long-term effects on our attention span and reduces our exposure to natural rhythms and light. For many of us, technology is so ingrained in our lives it is difficult to imagine living without it. We are not necessarily advocating for removing technology from our lives, just learning to live with it more consciously.

## The Role of Technology in Mental Health

Regarding severe mental illnesses, neurotechnology has been crucial in unraveling the brain mechanisms underlying some psychiatric disorders and in the creation of new and better drugs. This contributes to improving responses to existing treatments by targeting the most promising areas of the brain. The combination of electrophysiology and genetics on patients with different psychotic disorders, also ADHD, depression, and suicide, has made possible the discovery of specific biomarkers for early detection, risk assessment, and correlations with the severity of the disease. These findings have paved the way for predictive genetic testing and the creation of predictive analytical tools for a more accurate diagnosis. These combined neurotechnology analyses are a new hope for the millions of sufferers who have been historically underserved. They are additionally valuable for validated assessment and therapeutic monitoring agents. The correct choice of treatment, using an individualized method with organoid models, is a future predictable expansion given the problems present are related to a many-sided network of neuron cells and supporting cells from the cortex.

Information technology has made breakthroughs in the diagnosis and treatment of serious mental illnesses. Advances in neurotechnology, electronic health records, computer applications, mobile technologies, and the internet have revolutionized the screening and treatment for severe mental disorders such as schizophrenia, bipolar disorder, anxiety, depression, PTSD, and suicide. Artificial intelligence and machine learning have facilitated customization of treatment with personalized analytics, therapy innovations, and prediction tools. Technology has also expanded the number of participants that can be treated. The person having a mental health problem can choose from traditional therapeutic centers to digital treatment, in part to avoid the detection of having a mental problem or the inability to afford other options. The continuously decreasing cost of mobile technology and the extraordinary expansion of internet use has facilitated increasing treatment availability.

# CHAPTER 15

# Cultural Perspectives on Mental Wellness

Belief in spirits, superstitions, and fate are traditional explanations of mental illness in Greek and Asian cultures. A kap and drachma or other types of offerings may be used to perform cures. There is a strong "need to perform" at church to help recovery, and power may be sought from the priest or spiritual leader. Holy water, holy oil, crucifixes, incense, and candles lit at specific times can help facilitate recovery. Diet and special fasts have a role to play. Holy days and festivals have a strong spiritual significance in defining the patient's behavior in times of illness. Even in established Western societies, ethnic minority groups seem to find belonging in their culture's traditional concepts of fate and destiny. In the context of traditional views of national identity and resistance against Western colonization, spirit-worship and belief in old traditions may influence successful adjustment in a new culture. Family and community may guide old psychiatric methods reframing problems in the context of magical beliefs, even for Westernized generations living in Western societies.

Different cultures view mental illness in different ways. For instance, in many African and Caribbean cultures, there are strong stigmas attached to mental illness. Consequently, some members of these communities may be reluctant to talk about their problem. Indeed, when they receive help, it is often through the church rather than more traditional forms of Western medicine, such as the GP or a psychiatrist. Conversely, Asian and Greek cultures tend to view mental illness in a more spiritual or traditional way, associating their condition with fate, bad weather, the will of God, or ill fortune from the black arts or black magic, and only sometimes with anger, envy, or the worshiping of false gods. They are likely to seek both medical treatment and help from a traditional healer or spiritual guidance, as well as recognizing the importance of the church in helping them through their illness.

*Exploring Diverse Approaches*

Exercise can be very effective in the prevention and treatment of mental health issues. Running, weight lifting, hiking, and a variety of other physical activities have been shown to be of benefit. Vigorous exercise generally triggers the body to release endorphins and other chemicals that help manage pain, stress, and anxiety. Moderate exercise can improve mood, making a person feel at greater ease in their body. The distraction from daily life inherent in focusing on a physical activity is an added benefit, taking a person's mind off their daily worries. While most types of exercise can offer these mood management benefits, different types of exercise emphasize different components of mental health.

Mental health is a complex issue, and a variety of methods have proven effective in achieving and maintaining mental wellness. Some people begin their journey toward mental health by seeking traditional psychotherapy or by taking medication prescribed by a doctor. Other effective methods focus on improving physical health.

Still, others may seek solace in their faith or religious traditions or do extensive volunteer work to link up with others in the community and build a sense of purpose and satisfaction. Every person engaging in a journey toward mental health needs to find the path that works best for them, recognizing that other people are doing the same and that their preference may not be the same.

# CHAPTER 16

# The Future of Mental Wellness

In conclusion, we want to stress the importance of thinking systemically about mental health. This view revolves around the idea that many systems - from the physiological to the social - affect the health of the brain. Systems can enhance the brain's health, allowing it to serve as an efficient emotional immune system, protecting against and helping to recover from negative situations. Systems can also harm the brain's health, making the brain a liability, susceptible to mood disorders and mental illnesses. As a result, the mind should be thought of as a national asset and protected through mental wellness strategies that include things like mind-healthy neighborhoods, much like we protect other valuable assets through such strategies as national security or public health interventions. Indeed, going forward, mental wellness initiatives might take lessons from malign big problems, such as climate change or poverty, and embrace big solutions that tend to the mind. What we've learned in writing The Healthy Mind Blueprint suggests that with the right overall plan, it is possible for a population united in purpose to create a happy, thriving, and healthy nation by designing efficient systems that up-end the drive to accumulate unlimited wealth in exchange for creating uncommon amounts of wellness - a subject that we will turn to in the next blog book.

As we come to the end of our journey through The Healthy Mind Blueprint, we hope you've come away with a better understanding of mental wellness in general, recognize the integral role it plays in fostering overall health and increasing longevity, and are ready to prioritize your emotional health. We've discussed the consequences of untreated mental health disorders and their underlying mechanisms, particularly stress. We've recommended lifestyle changes and habits, from food choices to sleep habits, as a way to strengthen the mind and reduce stress. We've explored how the natural environment can foster better mental health and have discussed popular and effective approaches - from yoga and karate to herbs and acupuncture. We've looked closely at an innovative model of mental wellness aimed at identifying and mobilizing the strength of neighborhoods as a health intervention. Finally, we've traced the effects strengthening inner resources of the mind - promoting balance and creating a strong sense of meaning and purpose - can have on overall health.

*Innovations and Trends*

Recently, DeGroff, Schoonover, and Bauer described a movement within primary care training to adopt a preventive mental health approach that involves recognition, screening, assessment, brief intervention, treatment, and when appropriate, referral of eating disorders. Despite the value of these specified approach variables in both health and mental health domains, there are almost no studies that explore what students in primary occupational health training exercise experience and learn. The purpose of this innovative educational initiative was to address this change. Preliminary outcomes that demonstrate how students in primary care training communicate with, assess, intervene, and refer in these situations are presented.

In recent years, there has been an exponential growth in research and popular media on healthy minds and the prevention of mental health problems using different means, movements, or strategies. The adoption of strategies within different populations – within healthcare, educational, and developmental systems, across the workplace, and among the general public – illustrates social trends emphasizing personal and collective well-being, mental wellness, and the positive, by contrast to the healing of the negative. In this chapter, we share several new directions and innovations that have been generated from this trend.